Chapter 1

What is eating plant-based? To keep it simple, eating plant-based is defined as eating only foods that derive from a plant source. This means absolutely no animal sources of protein as ingredients. That's "plant-based." Plant-based is often referred to as vegan.

I want you to start thinking of this journey as an adventure in terms of what you can now enjoy as opposed to a long list of what you can no longer eat.

This is in no way a comprehensive list, but it will give you an idea of what "whole, plant-based foods" you can eat (getting started):

- Beans
- Potatoes
- Peas
- Rice
- Nuts
- Seeds
- Zucchini
- Squash
- Fruit – all varieties
- Avocado
- Mushrooms
- Tomato
- Oatmeal
- Cabbage
- Cauliflower
- Broccoli
- Collard greens
- Kale

- Swiss chard
- Spinach
- Romaine lettuce
- Bell peppers
- Jalapeno peppers
- Onions
- Corn
- Cucumber
- Olives
- Quinoa
- Eggplant
- Whole wheat pasta

Now that you have an idea of some basic plant-based foods, let's talk about tools that will help you in the kitchen as you embark on this wonderful journey of becoming a plant-based boss. As you progress along this journey, the number of "tools" you will need and use will be determined by your eating style, personal fitness or health goals, and personal preferences.

Here are my Top 10:

1. Blender (1000 watts or more)
2. Cutting board – various sizes and types
3. High-quality chef's knife
4. Food processor
5. Measuring utensils – all sizes
6. Spiralizer
7. Glass jars with caps – multiple sizes
8. Stainless steel cookware
9. Nut bag
10. Dehydrator

Bonus Tool:

1. Juicer

Chapter 2

Why Should I Eat Plant-Based?

Before we start answering all your plant-based "survival" questions, I want to tell you my story. This is a story about why I choose to eat plant-based (and how eating plant-based transformed my life and can do the same for you).

Let's start with my eating habits. I grew up eating the standard American diet (processed foods that were high in fat, high in sugar, and had plenty of salt). In the small town where I grew up and the area where I lived, fresh plant-based foods were not always readily available. This contributed to my nutritional habits (or lack thereof). I lived a very active and sport-driven lifestyle. Because of this activity, I appeared to be quite healthy. The issue was, I didn't realize that my eating habits were unhealthy and would eventually catch up to me.

Fast forward from my childhood/teenage years to college. Nothing about my diet really changed. Though I gained some weight in college, I didn't overanalyze my diet. My thought process was, "Everyone gains weight in college, right?" So life continued. I graduated from college, got married, and we decided to start a family.

Throughout my pregnancy, I continued to eat the standard American diet. By the time I gave birth, I weighed 211 pounds. Still, nothing drastic changed about the way I ate. After all, the way I ate was the "norm." I would, however, occasionally go on a "lose weight diet" and have some success. Plus, during this time of life, I was playing semiprofessional basketball. So yet again, because of my active lifestyle (and occasional dieting), I appeared to be healthy.

A few years later, during my second pregnancy, my first red flag (concerning my diet) appeared in the form of gestational diabetes. It was an emotional and scary experience. Not only did I fear for my quality of life but also for the life of my unborn child. However, after my delivery, the prediabetes was gone, my daughter was healthy, and although I had put on some weight, I appeared to be quite healthy. Again, nothing about my eating habits changed.

Nearly a year and half later, my 31 years of nutritional choices finally caught up to me. I was diagnosed with pre-diabetes and I was overweight. Honestly, I felt as though I had received a death sentence. You see, my grandmother, who had been battling and suffering through 20 years of diabetes, strokes, and kidney problems (as well as other diabetes-related issues), had recently passed away. All I could think about was that my life would end the way hers had. I believed my quality of life would slowly diminish, as I had seen my grandmother's health and overall wellbeing diminish over time. It was a very difficult and trying time in my life. Depression, stress, and worry consumed me.

The advice I received provided no comfort. Basically, I was told to avoid sweets (and other high-carb foods) and that when the time came, the proper medication would be provided. That simply wasn't good enough for me! That is when my "plant-based boss" pursuit began!

I was able to switch from a standard American diet of animal protein and processed side dishes to a plant-based diet. Plant-based (vegan) nutrition completely reversed my prediabetes, and I lost over 50 pounds in the process. In addition to the reversal of diabetes and the major weight loss, I had more energy and a better focus and outlook. My skin looks amazing, my brain is less foggy, my hair is growing and healthier than it was before, and my recovery time after exercise or sports is incredible. Plus, a plant-based diet is delicious!

As a trainer and coach, I've had the pleasure of seeing a plant-based diet make great health changes in the lives of others. Take my mom, Elzora; in 2017, she was having issues with an extremely low and irregular heartbeat. She had recently been hospitalized (due to stroke-like symptoms and an irregular heartbeat) and was told that she should see a cardiologist soon. Her cardiologist gave her a heart monitor so he could track the irregularities. He also scheduled her for a stress test that would take place three weeks after her initial visit to the doctor.

For the next three weeks, my mom followed a plant-based diet (80% of the time) and added in some walking. When she reported for her stress test, not only were her numbers great, but her heartbeat irregularities had disappeared!

Plants have so much power; you just have to eat them and find out! Plants truly rock!

Chapter 3

Let's Talk Mindset

First, if you're reading this "How to Eat Plant-Based Like a Boss" book, congrats! Your mindset has already changed and you are open to – or curious about – change. Mindset is one of the most important factors you will have to conquer on your eating-plant-based journey. Some people will support you, but there will be just as many (if not more) people who will not support you. Having a strong mindset, a different mindset from what you've always known or thought, is going to be key.

Take my childhood. I grew up eating your traditional soul-food dishes. You know, macaroni and cheese, neck bones and rice, bar-b-que ribs, collard greens with pork, fried fish and cheese grits, etc. The list could truly go on. That's what we ate. It was "normal." In fact, if you didn't eat those dishes, you were labeled as different. You were also on the receiving end of jokes. I can recall only one family member who was "different." The reason this person was different was because they enjoyed activities like yoga, exercised a lot, ate a ton of salads and veggies, and did not eat MEAT. Doesn't sound so far-fetched nowadays, but in my family (and many families like it), not eating meat was unheard of.

Now, because everyone in my family ate a standard American diet, I honestly didn't know what it meant to be vegetarian, let alone vegan or plant-based. But back to the point of this story: strong mindset. This family member was constantly answering questions, defending their dietary choices, and withstanding ridicule because of the way they ate. Can you imagine having your dietary choices become the major topic of conversation at every family function and gathering? And not just a topic of discussion but often a topic to poke fun at or make jokes about. However, because of their strong mindset, this family member never wavered. They continued to fill their plate with veggies and fruits … and they did so with a smile.

The point I'm making here is that you will undoubtedly face adversity, whether it's with family, at a restaurant, at a social event, or while traveling. But, rest assured, this adversity is temporary! Once you begin to eat plant-based like a boss, going to restaurants is no longer a stressful experience, being around family and social events becomes fun, knowing what to say when you're asked certain questions about the way you eat becomes automatic, and traveling is one of the greatest adventures you will get to experience. It all starts with your mindset! And, again, I congratulate you because you (your mindset) are either already there or on the way.

A huge part of your mindset shift is having an open mind. So, choose to be open-minded! You must be willing to try something new, eat something you have never heard of or seen, go to restaurants you've never visited, and cook foods you have never cooked before (in ways you have never used them).

There are thousands of different types of plants (fruits and vegetables). Never allow someone to say that eating plant-based is too restrictive, that there are not enough choices, or that you're going to get bored. The truth is, the options are limitless and the choices abound. It's up to you to have an open mind and to try them … mindset is key!

Chapter 4

Let's Talk Milk and Cheese

There are a variety of alternatives to your standard animal-protein-based milk. There are almond, cashew, soy, rice, banana, and coconut milks, to name a few. There are also a variety of flavors. The most popular flavors are vanilla, chocolate, sweetened, and unsweetened. Depending on where you live, you may have to go to a health food store to purchase the different varieties of non-dairy milk, but most of them can be found in your regular grocery store.

With so many choices, it can seem overwhelming to decide which milk you want to purchase. Remember to have an open mind and try out a few to determine your favorite.

The second option for non-dairy milk is to make your own. To make your own plant-based milk, you need a nut milk bag, your ingredient of choice (whether it's nuts, banana, or coconut), a blender, and spring water. I have a recipe for cashew milk in the recipe section if you prefer to take that route.

Just like a person can purchase non-dairy vegan milk, they can also purchase non-dairy vegan sliced cheese options from their local grocery stores. There are a plethora of choices. I suggest buying a few and trying them out. If you are looking for a parmesan cheese replacement, try nutritional yeast. I add it to salads, pastas, and dressings. It's also a handy ingredient to have around for many recipes.

You can also make your own cheese sauce. I've included two cheese sauce recipes in the recipe chapters. Enjoy them and make them your own.

Remember what I said about being open-minded.

Chapter 5

Let's Talk Meat and Protein

Let's take some time to discuss what tends to be one of the most important conversations I have with people when it comes to eating plant-based: meat. Common questions that you will encounter are: "How can you not eat meat?" and "What do you possibly eat instead of meat?" I believe this is one of the most frequent and common topics because, when I was a meat eater, I built my meals around meat. That's true for most meat eaters. Think about it: Meat is always the star. It is always the focal point.

Think about how most dishes are defined and named: by the meat they contain. For example, take the popular item fish and cheese grits. Fish is the meat around which the meal is built, and it's also mentioned first. Another example is fast food chains' menu options; look at the way the meals are written, with options like "sausage, egg, and biscuit" or "bacon, egg, and cheese." The stars in these cases are sausage and bacon, with the co-star being eggs.

This concept of the meat being the star doesn't apply just to fast food chains. Think about some common lunch items you can purchase from a deli or make at home: a ham and cheese sandwich, a chicken Caesar salad, and beef empanadas. All the meals begin with the meat. Meat is the star.

When you start eating plant-based like a boss, you must completely flip that idea upside down and inside out. No longer is meat the star of your plate. Now what you once considered an afterthought, or just a side item (in some cases, nonexistent) is the focal point or star of your plate. You will begin to build your meal around your veggies, potatoes, beans, rice, and fruit.

This is why spending some time talking about meat alternatives is important. When you start to build these meals, your first strategy will be to think about your meals the "old way." I want you to be able to take the old way of meal building and "plant-base it."

Take one of those examples I just mentioned: the sausage, egg, and biscuit sandwich. It's actually pretty simple to "plant-base it." Use a meat alternative, such as vegan sausage, which you will see referred to as mock meats, and combine it with a slice of melted vegan cheese as well as with scrambled vegan eggs. Put those plant-based alternatives on a dairy-free, animal protein-free biscuit, and boom: You just plant-based your first meal! Sitting on your plate is a delicious vegan sausage, vegan scrambled eggs, and vegan sliced cheese biscuit sandwich!

Congrats, boss!

Now, you will find that some people who eat plant-based do not advocate for or eat mock meats. If you choose to fall into that category because you want to consume plant-based, whole foods that are unprocessed, you'll find the effort is just as easy. You'll still take that original concept of meat as your star and flip it. It will just look a bit different. So, let's say you decide to have a taco night. Typically, you would have ground beef, cheese, lettuce, tomato, and onion. Instead, as a plant-based boss, you can make walnut taco meat and cashew-based cheese sauce (or use nutritional yeast). Then you'd add lettuce, tomatoes, onions, and tortillas. You just plant-based another meal! I could go on, but I'm sure you get the point. Plant-basing your meals is a pretty simple process. It all comes back to mindset and open-mindedness.

Here is a list of popular plant-based mock meats. These can be helpful during your transition period. If you've already transitioned, they could serve as quick alternatives or even as weekly treats. Remember, instead of thinking about meat first and building a meal around it, flip the concept; think either alternative swap and build, or pick a side and surround it with delicious and nutritious fruits and vegetables.

Here's a list of common mock meats:

- Tempeh
- Tofu
- Seitan
- Store-bought chicken alternatives
- Store-bought beef alternatives
- Store-bought fish alternatives
- Store-bought sausage alternatives
- Store-bought cold cut alternatives

- Store-bought bacon alternatives

When shopping for vegan meat alternatives, you'll find that the frozen food section, produce section, and dairy section are your best bet. If you're ever in doubt, ask someone to help you.

If you choose to make your "meat," here are some options:

- Walnut meat

  o Similar to a ground meat crumble. (I've included a recipe in Chapter 13).

- Jackfruit

  o Great as a pulled meat alternative. Tastes great with barbecue sauce.

- Mushrooms

  o Portobello mushrooms are pretty easy to work with.

  o They taste great grilled (as "steaks") too.

  o They can also be blended for tasty sauces and gravies.

- Lentils and beans

  o Excellent texture for homemade burgers.

- Cauliflower

  o Great alternative to traditional meat chicken wings. You can use the same process that you use to make chicken wings and simply apply it to the cauliflower florets. (I've included a recipe in Chapter 13).

Now that you have plenty of ways to tackle "meat" in your dishes, let's talk protein. Often, when people think about protein, they immediately think of meat. When people hear "plant-based eating," they still think of protein but mostly with curiosity about how someone who doesn't eat meat gets their protein.

This will be one of the most common questions you will be asked by family, friends, and even strangers once they find out that you are plant-based. The question will be: "Where do you get your protein?" Take a deep breath and tell them that protein is found in every fruit or vegetable, particularly green vegetables. In fact, in my experience, most green vegetables that I regularly consume have just as much, if not more, protein than common meats. Don't believe me? Conduct an internet search on the protein found in peas, broccoli, kale, and spinach. Then compare it to the protein in common meats. Wowzer!

In addition to fruits and vegetables, you can get protein from beans, nuts, seeds, protein powders, protein bars, and mock meats. A ton of options are available. Don't stress it. Just eat a variety of foods and the protein will take care of itself.

Chapter 6

Let's Talk Desserts

Who has a sweet tooth? I do. I do. Let's talk about the sweet stuff! Here's the good news: You don't have t o give up sweets or stop having your favorite desserts. There are plant-based options to satisfy those cravings! Yay!

In chapter 11, I've listed some common alternatives you can use to plant-base your favorite recipes. The fun part of being plant-based with a sweet tooth is the wealth of recipes you try (and taste).

Cakes, ice cream, pies, muffins, cookies, and even fat bombs are some of my go-to plant-based options whenever I have a sweet tooth. Even items like pancakes and smoothies can satisfy a "dessert craving." In the recipe sections, I've included a recipe for pancakes and smoothies.

If you aren't into the "making it yourself" concept, there's always the restaurant option. In the beginning, and even now after years of being plant-based, I enjoy visiting restaurants that specialize in vegan desserts. I've had every – and I do mean every – type of dessert while out exploring different restaurants. Yummy!

Lastly, in your popular food markets, there are usually quite a few vegan-friendly alternatives to your favorite non-vegan desserts. Look around and try them out. You'll find something that you enjoy.

There are too many store-bought "sweets" options to list, but here are a few:

- Dark chocolate
- Granola bars
- Most cereals
- Oreos
- Unfrosted Pop-Tarts

- Most candy

Chapter 7

Let's Talk Restaurants and Traveling

The first thing you should do when you decide what restaurant you will dine at is visit the restaurant's website and find its nutritional facts. Most restaurants offer this information. Look for vegan-friendly options. This will ensure that you are prepared; you will know what you can and cannot order and what your various options are. If the restaurant does not have a fully functioning nutrition link that provides this information, don't be afraid to ask your server. Most times – and I say most times – the items on the sides menu will be your go-to items, as many sides are plant-based.

Preparation of items is something you must become comfortable asking your server about. Typically, restaurants will sauté, steam, or cook the vegetables in butter, dairy, added meat, and animal protein broths. If this is the case, mention to your server that you are vegan and explain that you do not want any of the aforementioned items used in the preparation of your food.

Of course, you can also have salad as an entrée. A great restaurant meal could be a garden salad with no meat, no cheese, and no croutons, and with Italian dressing. Add a baked potato, a little light seasoning, and steamed or sautéed vegetables without butter, and congratulations – you just survived a night out at a restaurant. Now, that was just a sample meal, but between the restaurant's nutritional link with the ingredient breakdown and the vegan/vegetarian sections on restaurant menus, you'll have options, so don't worry.

Traveling can be tricky at first; where you're going matters quite a bit. If you're traveling in the US, you can approach your diet in the same way you do at restaurants – seek side items and don't be bashful when it comes to asking questions. If you're going out of the country, some safe bets could be fruit, vegetables in their raw state, and French fries.

If you're cruising, visiting an all-inclusive resort, or flying, call ahead and make them aware that you are plant-based (vegan) and would like to know if they have vegan options (and what those options are). Always plan ahead! This will decrease any anxiety and make the trip worthwhile. Another must-do when traveling to different cities, states, and even countries is to use vegan restaurant locator apps and websites. Know where the good spots are ahead of time. Not only is it fun to try various cuisines, but your taste buds will be happy, too.

Chapter 8

Let's Talk Social Events and Holidays

In the beginning, eat before you go. In fact, sometimes, even after the beginning, eat before you go. Because here's the deal: You don't want to put yourself into a situation in which you're hungry and there's nothing "plant-based" for you to eat. When I plan to eat beforehand, I find it thoughtful to let the host know that they do not need to prepare anything special for me.

Trust me, this is a big help. You don't want to be at a family gathering or social event where the host has made food especially for you and you don't eat it because you have eaten beforehand. They will notice, trust me.

Now, if the host insists on prepping a dish for you, let them. They may surprise you with something delicious that you have never had before. Plus, it's nice to be supported. Thank them for their thoughtfulness.

Another way you can approach social events and holidays is to bring a dish. Depending on the social event or the openness of your family, you may want to bring enough for just you. If your family and friends are interested and supportive, bring enough to share. Plant-based boss tip: Bring dishes that you make well and that taste incredible. In the recipe section, I've included a sweet and spicy cauliflower wings recipe and a Mexican black bean salad dish that crowds tend to enjoy. This could be a great opportunity to turn others into plant-based bosses, too!

You will notice that as more people learn you are plant-based, your dishes will be welcomed and, in some cases, even requested at events. Get ready to change the world. ☺

Chapter 9

Let's Talk Food Labels

Please read the food labels of any and all food that comes out of a package. Don't just read the front of the box and make your "plant-based" decision based on that. Turn that package over, look at the ingredients, and scan them. Now, I'm not going to go over the obvious no-no's, such as milk, eggs, cheese, cream, chicken, beef, pork, turkey, etc. I want to list some of the more hidden ones that you might not be aware are derived from animal sources. Here are a few:

- Gelatin
- Casein
- Whey
- Lard
- Lactose

If in doubt, don't buy the product, or first conduct an internet search of the unknown ingredient. What you discover will surprise you.

Chapter 10

Let's Talk Supplements, Spices, Seasonings, and Herbs

Please allow me to remind you that I am not a doctor, nutritionist, or physician. I cannot heal, cure, or diagnose you with or of anything.

A common question I get is: "What kind of supplements do you take?" Here's a list of supplements that I either use personally or that are used by people I know:

- Daily multi-vitamin (make sure it's vegan-friendly)
- Dried greens powder
- Trace minerals
- Vitamin B12
- Vitamin D
- Sea moss
- Herbal tea
- Black seed oil
- Turmeric
- Chlorella
- Spirulina

Plant-based boss tip: Always remember to conduct your own research. Do what's best for you and your health.

Why do my plant-based dishes taste so great? The easy answer is flavor, flavor, and more flavor! One key to eating plant-based and not "looking back" is adding flavor to your dishes. Truth is, the meat dishes that many feel they simply can't give up, are their "favorite foods" because of the seasonings, herbs, and spices, not because of the meat itself. Trust me. You are about to embark on a delicious new journey and plants with the perfect flavor combinations are the star.

Below I've listed some of my go to herbs, spices, and seasonings:

- Pink Himalayan Salt
- Black Pepper
- Cayenne Pepper
- Garlic
- Onion
- Celery
- Paprika
- Cumin
- Oregano
- Basil
- Parsley
- Curry

Take some time in the kitchen and really develop the flavors that fit your taste. Once you have mastered the flavors you like, putting together delicious plant-based meals is simple.

Chapter 11

What Can I Use Instead?

Below I've listed a few more alternatives that you can use in place of animal-based sources in your dishes.

Alternatives List

☐ **Meat**

- Tofu
- Tempeh
- Seitan
- Soy-based meats
- Veggie burgers

☐ **Cheese**

- Nutritional yeast
- Cashew cheese
- Store products

☐ **Dairy**

- Almond milk
- Cashew milk
- Soy milk
- Rice milk
- Banana milk

☐ **Substitutes for eggs**

- ¼ cup of applesauce = 1 egg
- 1 tablespoon ground flax seeds mixed with 3 tablespoons of water = 1 egg
- Store products = vegan eggs

- **Substitutes for flour**
  - Oats
  - Whole wheat
  - Almond flour
  - Coconut flour
- **Substitutes for sugar (regular sugar is vegan)**
  - Coconut sugar
  - Raw sugar
  - Blended Medjool dates
  - Agave nectar
  - Monk fruit (low-carb friendly)
  - Stevia (low-carb friendly)
- **Substitutes for butter**
  - Store-bought vegan butter
  - Mashed avocado

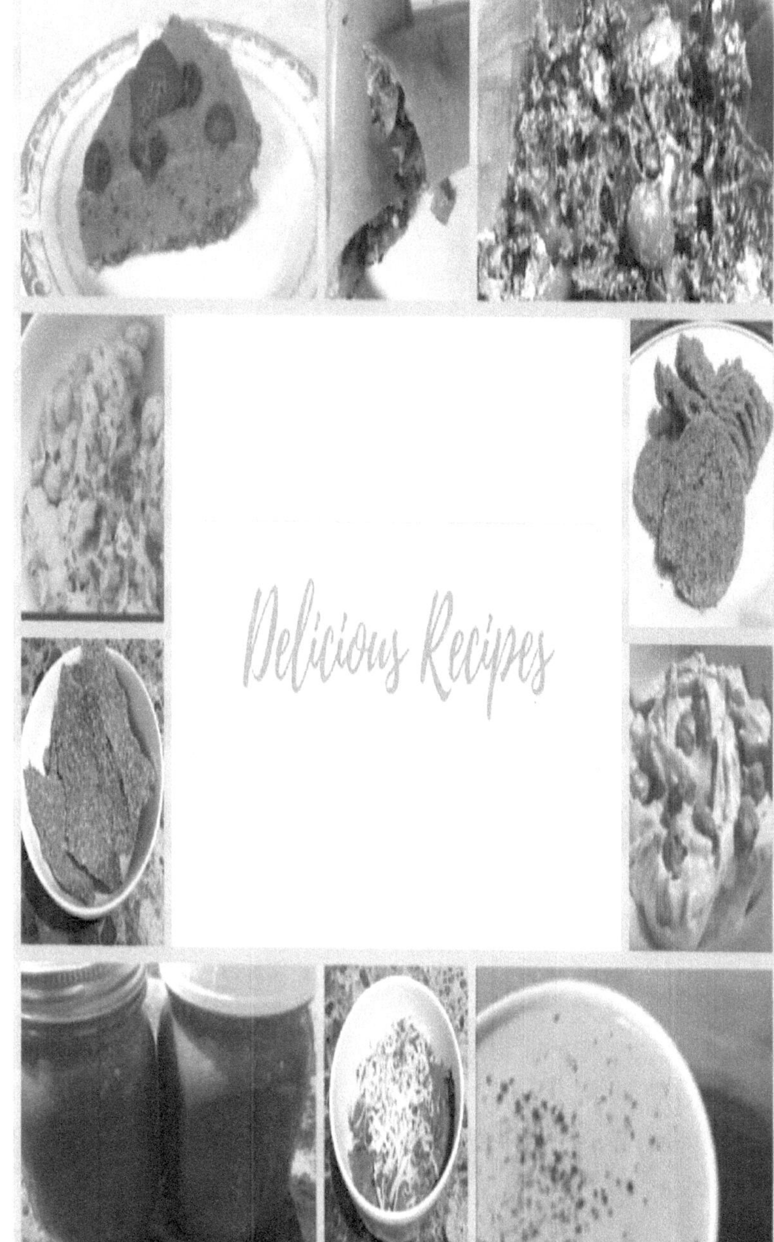
Delicious Recipes

Chapter 12

Plant-Based Breakfast Recipes

1. Blueberry Banana Pancakes

☐ **Ingredients**

- 1 Cup Unsweetened Almond Milk (or non-dairy milk of your choice)
- 2 Bananas
- ½ Cup Blueberries
- 1½ Cups Whole Wheat Flour
- 1 Teaspoon Cinnamon
- ½ Tablespoon Coconut sugar
- Dash of Salt
- 1 Teaspoon Baking Powder
- Vegan Butter or Non-Stick Cooking Spray

☐ **Tools**

- Blender
- Pan

☐ **Method**

» Blend bananas and ¼ cup blueberries with non-dairy milk.

» Combine wet and dry ingredients in mixing bowl. Mix batter. (If too thin, add more flour. If too thick, add more non-dairy milk.)

» Allow to settle.

» Use vegan butter or non-stick spray on pan.

Fry on hot pan or griddle 1–3 minutes on each side (depending on
» thickness).

Before flipping one side, sprinkle remaining blueberries evenly through
» each pancake.

» Enjoy.

2. Banana Chia Seed Pudding

☐ **Ingredients**

- 3 Tablespoons Chia Seeds
- 1½ Cups Coconut Milk (or other non-dairy milk)
- 1½ Bananas
- 1 Tablespoon Agave Nectar
- 1 Teaspoon Cinnamon

☐ **Tools**

- Mason Jar (with lid)
- Blender

☐ **Method**

» Blend 1 banana and ½ coconut milk. Pour into mason jar.

» Cut ½ banana into slices.

» Combine all remaining ingredients into mason jar.

» Close cap.

» Shake until well mixed.

Refrigerate a minimum of 4–6 hours. (The longer it refrigerates, the
» thicker it becomes.)

3. Peanut Butter Chia Seed Pudding (Low-Carb Friendly)

☐ **Ingredients**

- 3 Tablespoons Chia Seeds
- 1½ Cups Cashew Milk (or other non-dairy milk)
- 1 Scoop Peanut Butter Protein Powder
- 2 Stevia Drops

☐ **Tools**

- Mason Jar (with lid)

☐ **Method**

» Combine all ingredients in mason jar.

» Close cap.

» Shake until well mixed.

Refrigerate a minimum of 4–6 hours (The longer it refrigerates, the
» thicker it becomes.)

4. Loaded Tofu Scramble (Low-Carb Friendly)

☐ **Ingredients**

- 1 Block Firm Tofu
- 2½ Cups Spinach
- ¼ Cup Diced Mushrooms
- ½ Diced Bell Pepper
- ½ Diced Onion
- ½ Cup Nutritional Yeast
- Store-Bought Vegan Cheese
- 2 Teaspoons Store-Bought Vegan Butter
- ¼ Cup Vegetable Broth
- 2 Teaspoons Garlic Powder
- Pink Himalayan Salt (to taste)
- Pepper (to taste)

☐ **Tools**

- Pan

☐ **Method**

» Remove excess liquid by pressing tofu with napkins or towel.

» Sauté onions and peppers in vegan butter for 1 minute.

» Stir in crumbled tofu. Cook for 3 minutes.

Add 3 tablespoons nutritional yeast and dry seasonings. Stir and cook for
» 1 minute.

» Continue to stir and add ¼ cup vegetable broth. Cook for 3 minutes.

» Add spinach. Stir and cook for 1 minute.

» Top with vegan cheddar cheese.

» Mix for 1 minute or until cheese is melted.

5. Coconut Pecan 'N Oatmeal (Low-Carb Friendly)

☐ **Ingredients**

- 1½ Cups Non-Dairy Milk (I use unsweetened coconut milk.)
- ½ Cup Hemp Seeds
- 1 Tablespoon Chia Seeds
- 1 Tablespoon Ground Flax Seed
- 1 Tablespoon Unsweetened Coconut Flakes
- 1 Teaspoon Cinnamon
- 3 Drops Stevia (more if you like it sweet)
- 2 Tablespoons Pecan Nut Butter

☐ **Tools**

- Pot
- Measuring Utensils

☐ **Method**

» Combine 1 cup non-dairy milk with all ingredients, except pecan nut butter.

» Boil and stir for 10 minutes under medium heat.

» Pour into bowl. Allow to settle 1–2 minutes.

» Top with pecan nut butter.

» Top with coconut flakes (optional).

» Enjoy!

Chapter 13

Plant-Based Lunch/Dinner Recipes

<u>6. Sweet and Spicy Cauliflower Wings</u>

☐ **Ingredients**
- ½ Cauliflower Head
- 1½ Cups Almond Milk
- 1 Cup Whole Wheat Flour
- Pink Himalayan Salt (to taste)
- Black Pepper (to taste)
- 1 Teaspoon Cumin
- 2 Teaspoons Garlic Powder
- 2 Teaspoons Onion Powder
- 1 Teaspoon Paprika
- 1 Bottle of Sweet BBQ Sauce
- 1 Tablespoon Hot Sauce (add more if you prefer spicier)
- 1 Tablespoon Vegan Butter
- ½ Tablespoon Agave Nectar

☐ **Tools**
- Baking Sheet
- Mixing Bowl
- Small Pot
- Parchment Paper

☐ **Method**

» Preheat oven to 450 degrees.

» To make batter: Mix almond milk, flour, and dry seasonings in mixing bowl until well blended. If too thick, add more milk; if too thin, add more flour.

» Wash and cut cauliflower into florets.

» Line baking sheet with parchment paper.

» Dip florets into batter. Shake off excess batter.

» Place dipped cauliflower florets onto parchment paper.

» To make sauce: In pot, combine butter, BBQ sauce, hot sauce, and agave nectar. Keep on medium to low heat and stir frequently.

» Bake for 25 minutes. Flip halfway through.

» Take cauliflower wings out of oven and coat with sweet and spicy sauce.

» Put wings back in oven for 15-20 minutes; flip halfway through. You want them crispy but not burnt, so watch them☺.

» Take them out and coat with more sauce.

» Let cool.

» Enjoy!

7. Barbecue Baked Tofu

Ingredients
- 1 Block Extra Firm Tofu
- 1 Tablespoon Coconut Oil
- 2 Tablespoons Vegan Butter (optional)
- 2 Teaspoons Garlic Powder
- 2 Teaspoons Onion Powder
- Pink Himalayan Salt (to taste)
- Black Pepper (to taste)
- BBQ Sauce of Choice

Tools
- Stove
- Baking Pan or Sheet

Method

» Open tofu package and drain liquid.

» Cut tofu into cubes. Cut evenly so it will cook evenly.

» Place cubes into mixing bowl. Pour coconut oil over cubes. Toss gently.

» Season with dry seasonings.

Add sauce and toss evenly. Allow to sit and absorb marinade for at least
» 30 minutes.

» Bake at 375 degrees for 20 minutes, then flip over for 10 minutes.

» Let cool a bit and add more sauce.

» Enjoy.

<u>8. Chickpea Tuna-Less Salad</u>

☐ **Ingredients**

- 2 Cups Cooked Chickpeas (canned chickpeas 19 oz.) drained and rinsed
- 1 Nori Wrap
- ¼ Cup Onions, Diced
- 2 Tablespoons Sweet Relish
- 1½ Tablespoons Dijon Mustard
- 1 Tablespoon Minced Garlic
- 2 Teaspoons Poultry Seasoning
- 1 Teaspoon Mustard Seed
- 1 Teaspoon Celery Seed
- ⅔ Cup Vegan Mayo
- 1 Tablespoon Apple Cider Vinegar
- 1 Teaspoon Black Pepper
- Pink Himalayan Salt (to taste)

☐ **Tools**

- Food Processor
- Blender or Grinder
- Mixing Bowl

☐ **Method**

» Use a blender or grinder to grind nori wrap.

» Mash chickpeas (keep chunky).

» Combine all ingredients in food processor.

» Pulse until combined (keep chunky).

» Pour into container/bowl.

» Refrigerate at least 30 minutes.

» Enjoy.

9. Macaroni and Cheese

☐ **Ingredients**

- ½ Box Macaroni Pasta
- 1 Cup Nutritional Yeast
- ¼ Onion, Diced
- 1 Tablespoon Mustard
- ½ Cup Vegetable Broth
- 1 Cup Non-Dairy Milk
- ½ Cup Water
- 1 Cup Vegan Shredded Cheddar Cheese (store-bought)
- ¼ Cup Vegan Butter (store-bought)
- 1 Tablespoon Italian Seasoning
- Black Pepper (to taste)
- Pink Himalayan Salt (to taste)
- Dash of Parsley

☐ **Tools**

- Pot
- Baking Pan
- Stove

☐ **Method**

» Boil pasta. Drain and rinse. Set aside.

» For cheese sauce:

On stove (warm temperature) – in pot, combine vegan butter, vegetable broth, water, non-dairy milk, mustard, onion, nutritional yeast, ½ cup vegan shredded cheese, pink Himalayan salt, and black pepper.

Stir until well blended and cheese is melted.

Combine cooked pasta with cheese sauce in mixing bowl. Stir until well

» mixed.

» Top with dash of pink Himalayan salt and parsley.

» Preheat oven to 350 degrees.

» In oven pan:

Grease baking pan with non-stick spray, vegan butter, or coconut oil.

Pour macaroni and cheese mixture into pan.

Top with ½ cup vegan shredded cheese.

Bake 15–20 minutes (until shredded cheese is melted).

» Enjoy.

10. Coconut Corn Chowder

☐ **Ingredients**

- 6 Cups Corn
- 2 Cubed Russet Potatoes (with skin on)
- 1 Cup Finely Chopped Spinach
- 2 Small Chopped Carrots
- 1 Medium Onion
- 1 Diced Red Bell Pepper
- 2 Cans Coconut Milk
- 1 Cup Vegetable Broth
- ½ Tablespoon Garlic Powder
- 1 Vegetable Bouillon Cube
- 1 Lemon, Squeezed
- 2 Teaspoons Parsley
- 1 Sheet of Nori
- Pink Himalayan Salt (to taste)

☐ **Tools**

- Pot

- Blender

□ **Method**

» Sautee onion and bell peppers.

» Add vegetables (carrots, potatoes, corn, and spinach).

» Stir until well blended under medium heat.

» Add liquids (coconut milk, vegetable broth, lemon juice).

» Allow to boil for 20 minutes.

» Use blender to grind nori sheet.

» Add nori to pot and stir well.

  Pour half mixture into blender (make sure to get good portion of veggies).

» Blend until smooth.

» Pour blended mixture back into pot.

» Add all dry seasonings.

» Continue to cook for 10–20 minutes (until potatoes are done).

» Allow to sit for 10 minutes.

» Enjoy.

11. Onion Chia Crackers (Low-Carb Friendly)

□ **Ingredients**

- 4 Tablespoons Chia Seeds
- 1 Tablespoon Onion Powder
- 1 Teaspoon Garlic Powder
- ¼ Teaspoon Pink Himalayan Salt
- ½ Teaspoon Black Pepper
- ½ Teaspoon Oregano
- 1 Tablespoon Vegetable Broth
- ½ Cup Water

□ **Tools**

- Dehydrator or Oven

□ **Method**

» Combine all dry ingredients in mixing bowl.

» Mix thoroughly.

» Combine all wet ingredients in mixing bowl.

» Mix thoroughly.

» Let sit for 1 minute.

» Spread (to desired thickness) onto dehydrator sheets or parchment paper. If cooking in oven: 3 hours, 200 degrees. Flip after 1.5 hours (depending

» on thickness).

» OR: 12–15 hours in dehydrator (depending on thickness).

12. Walnut Meat (Low-Carb Friendly)

☐ **Ingredients**

- 1 Cup Walnuts
- ¼ Medium Onion, Diced
- ½ Teaspoon Black Pepper
- ½ Teaspoon to 1 Teaspoon Pink Himalayan Salt (to taste)
- 1 Teaspoon Garlic Powder
- 1 Teaspoon Onion Powder
- 1 Teaspoon Poultry Seasoning
- ¼ Cup Vegetable Broth

☐ **Method**

» In food processor, combine all ingredients.

» Pulse until it looks like "ground meat."

» If enjoying raw, go ahead and enjoy.

» If enjoying cooked, sauté in pan 1–2 minutes under low heat.

» Enjoy.

<u>13. Chocolate Mug Cake (Low-Carb Friendly)</u>

☐ **Ingredients**

- 1 Scoop Chocolate Protein Powder (32 grams)
- ½ Teaspoon Baking Powder
- 1 Tablespoon Coconut Flour
- 1 Tablespoon Stevia
- 1 Tablespoon Vegan Butter
- ¼ Cup Unsweetened Applesauce
- ¼ Cup Unsweetened Almond Milk
- ¼ Teaspoon Vanilla Extract
- Chocolate Chips to Top (optional)

☐ **Tools**

- Coffee Mug
- Microwave

☐ **Method**

» Mix all dry ingredients in bowl.

» Melt butter and mix with all wet ingredients.

» Combine ingredients in coffee mug.

» Add chocolate chips (optional).

» Microwave for 60–75 seconds. (I used a 1000-watt microwave.)

» Allow to cool.

» Eat in mug or dump out of mug.

» Enjoy.

14. Peanut Butter Green Fat Bomb Bars

(Low-Carb Friendly)

☐ **Ingredients**

- 1 Cup Coconut Oil
- 1 Scoop Peanut Butter Protein Powder
- Handful Crushed Peanuts
- 1 Scoop Store-Bought Dried Greens Mix (green vegetable supplement powder) (optional)

☐ **Tools**

- Pot
- Stove
- Baking Molds

☐ **Method**

» On stove (medium heat), melt coconut oil.

» Mix in protein powder.

» Mix in greens powder.

» Add 2 drops stevia.

» Stir until well blended.

» Allow to cool slightly.

» Pour into molds.

» Place in freezer for 30 minutes to an hour.

» Enjoy.

15. Banana Caramel Nice Cream

☐ **Ingredients**

- 2½ Frozen Bananas
- 1 Tablespoon Vanilla Extract

- 1 Teaspoon Cinnamon
- 1 Tablespoon Agave Nectar
- 2–4 Medjool Dates
- Cinnamon Almonds (optional)

☐ **Tools**

- Blender

☐ **Method**

» Caramel Date Sauce – combine 4 Medjool dates and agave in blender (set aside).

» Combine all other ingredients in blender and blend. (It will be thick.)

» Pour Nice Cream in bowl. Top with "Caramel Date" sauce.

» Add cinnamon almonds on top (optional).

» Enjoy.

16. Chocolate Mousse (Low-Carb Friendly)

☐ **Ingredients**

- 2 Avocados
- 1 Tablespoon Cocoa Powder
- 1 Tablespoon Non-Dairy Milk
- 2 Teaspoons Vanilla Extract
- 4 Stevia Drops or 3 Tablespoons Agave Nectar (if using agave, it will not be low-carb)
- 1 Teaspoon Pink Himalayan Salt

☐ **Tools**

- Blender

☐ **Method**

» In bowl, use fork to smash avocados.

» Add to blender.

» Add wet ingredients (milk, vanilla extract, and agave).

» Add cacao powder and salt.

» Blend until "mousse" consistency.

17. Berry Banana Cream Pie

□ **Ingredients**

- ½ Cup Blueberries
- 1 Cup Strawberries
- 3 Bananas
- 2 Frozen Bananas
- 2 Cups Soaked Almonds
- 8 Medjool Dates
- 4 Teaspoons Cinnamon
- 2 Teaspoons Vanilla Extract
- 1 Tablespoon Agave Nectar

□ **Tools**

- Blender
- Baking Pan
- Food Processor

□ **Method**

» For Crust

In processor, pulse almonds, Medjool dates, cinnamon, and vanilla extract.

Flatten crust mixture into baking pan.

For Pie Filling

In blender, blend bananas, blueberries, strawberries, and agave nectar.

Blend until smooth but thick.

Pour filling into pie crust.

Top with cut strawberries, blueberries, and banana slices (optional).

Place in freezer for 1 hour.

Enjoy.

18. Chocolate Nutty Bar

□ **Ingredients**

- 1 Cup Nut Butter of Choice (Peanut Butter, Almond Butter, or Pecan

Butter)

- 2 Cups Raw Nuts (Almonds, Walnuts, Pecans)
- ½ Cup Coconut Oil
- ¼ Cup Coconut Flakes (optional)
- 1 Tablespoon Chia Seeds
- 2 Scoops Protein Powder (I use Garden of Life)
- 3 Medjool Dates

Tools

- Processor
- Baking Pan

Method

» Combine all ingredients in food processor.

» Pulse until "thick" and combined.

» Spoon mix into baking pan.

» Place in refrigerator for 2-4 hours.

» Cut into bars.

» Enjoy

Chapter 15

Plant-Based Sauces, Dips, and Dressing Recipes

19. Raw Nacho Cheese Sauce

☐ **Ingredients**

- 1 Cup Cashews
- ¼ Medium Onion
- 1 Teaspoon Cayenne Pepper
- 1 Teaspoon Pink Himalayan Salt
- 1 Teaspoon Italian Seasoning
- ½ Cup Vegetable Broth (add more if too thick)
- ½ Cup Nutritional Yeast
- ¼ Medium Bell Pepper

☐ **Tools**

- Blender

☐ **Method**

» Combine all ingredients except nutritional yeast in blender.

» Blend until smooth.

» Add nutritional yeast.

» Blend.

» If too thick, add ¼ cup more vegetable broth (until desired thickness).

» Enjoy!

20. Spicy Avocado Dill Dressing (Low-Carb Friendly)

Ingredients

- ½ Avocado
- 1 Tablespoon Coconut Oil
- 1 Teaspoon Apple Cider Vinegar
- ½ Lemon, Squeezed
- ½ Teaspoon Fresh Dill
- ½ Teaspoon Oregano
- ¼ Teaspoon Onion Powder
- ¼ Teaspoon Garlic Powder
- ¼ Teaspoon Cayenne Pepper

Tools

- Blender

Method

» Combine all wet ingredients with avocado.

» Blend.

» Add all dry ingredients.

» Blend.

» Enjoy.

21. Mango Salsa

Ingredients

- ¼ Onion, Diced
- ¼ Bell Pepper (Red or Orange), Diced
- "Palm Amount" Cilantro, Diced
- Jalapenos, Diced (optional – if you want it spicy)
- 1 Large Mango Cut into Chunks
- 1 Tablespoon Lime Juice
- 1 Tablespoon Lemon Juice
- 1 Teaspoon Black Pepper
- Dash of Pink Himalayan Salt

Tools

- None

□ **Method**

» Combine all ingredients in bowl.

» Mix evenly.

» Enjoy.

22. Lemon Vinaigrette (Low-Carb Friendly)

□ **Ingredients**

- 1 Tablespoon Olive Oil
- 1 Lemon, Squeezed
- 3 Teaspoons Italian Seasoning
- Pink Himalayan Salt (to taste)
- ¼ Teaspoon Black Pepper

□ **Tools**

- Bowl
- Whisk

□ **Method**

» Combine all ingredients in bowl.

» Mix evenly.

» Enjoy.

23. Spicy Peanut Dressing

□ **Ingredients**

- ¼ Cup Peanuts
- 1 Tablespoon Agave Nectar
- 2 Tablespoons Vegetable Broth
- ¼ Tablespoon Apple Cider Vinegar
- 1 Teaspoon Coconut Oil
- 1 Teaspoon Black Pepper and Pink Himalayan Salt
- 2 Teaspoons Cayenne Pepper

□ **Tools**

- Blender

□ **Method**

» Blend peanuts with vegetable broth and apple cider vinegar. Combine and whisk in bowl. Blend peanuts with coconut oil and dry
» seasonings.
» Enjoy.

Chapter 16

Plant-Based Green Smoothie and Juice Recipes

24. Blueberry Green Blast

□ **Ingredients**

- 1 Cup Spinach
- 1 Medium Frozen Banana
- 1 Cup Frozen or Fresh Blueberries or Fresh
- 2 Teaspoons Cinnamon
- 8–12 Ounces Unsweetened Vanilla Almond Milk (depending on desired thickness)

□ **Tools**

- Blender

□ **Method**

» Combine all ingredients in blender.

» Blend until smooth.

» Enjoy.

25. Chocolate Dream (Low-Carb Friendly)

□ **Ingredients**

- 1 Scoop Chocolate Protein Powder (look for 1 net carb or less)
- 1 Tablespoon Chia Seeds
- 2 Drops Stevia
- ½ Cup Ice

- 10 Ounces Unsweetened Coconut Milk
- 1 Serving Perfect Keto Chocolate MCT Oil Powder or 1 Tablespoon Cocoa Powder (add additional 1-2 drops of stevia if you choose this option)

□ **Tools**
- Blender

□ **Method**

» Combine all ingredients in blender.

» Blend.

» Enjoy!

26. Pear Green Juice

□ **Ingredients**
- 4 Cups Organic Spinach
- 10 Grams Ginger
- 1 Bunch Organic Celery
- 4 Organic Pears
- 1 Organic Lemon

□ **Tools**
- Juicer
- Strainer
- Cutting Knife

□ **Method**

» Clean and prep fruits and vegetables.

» Put through juicer.

» Use strainer to pour juice into container.

» Enjoy.

27. Kickin' Celery Juice

□ **Ingredients**

- ½ Bunch Organic Celery
- ½ Cucumber
- 3 Apples
- 1 Organic Lemon
- 10 Grams Ginger
- 5 Grams Turmeric

Tools

- Juicer
- Strainer
- Cutting Knife

Method

» Clean and prep fruits and vegetables.

» Put through juicer.

» Use strainer to pour juice into container.

» Enjoy.

Chapter 17

Plant-Based Salad Recipes

<u>28. Mexican Black Bean Salad</u>

☐ Ingredients

- ½ Can Black Beans (drained)
- ½ Can Corn (drained)
- ½ to ¾ Can Garlic Basil Diced Tomato (If you are a tomato fan, go with ¾ instead of ½ ù)
- 1 Medium Avocado
- ¼ Diced White Onion
- ½ Bell Pepper
- 2 Teaspoons Garlic Powder
- ½ Lime, Squeezed
- Pink Himalayan Salt (to taste)
- Black Pepper (to taste)

☐ Tools

- Mixing Bowl

☐ Method

» Smash avocado in mixing bowl using fork.

» Add onions, bell pepper, garlic, salt, and pepper.

» Mix thoroughly.

» Add black beans and corn.

» Mix thoroughly.

» Add diced tomatoes.

» Mix.

» Top with lime juice.

» Enjoy!

29. Cheesy Kale Salad (Low-Carb Friendly)

- ☐ **Ingredients**
  - 3 Cups Kale
  - 8 Cherry Tomatoes (sliced in half)
  - ½ Avocado
  - ¼ Sliced Onion
  - 1 Lemon, Squeezed
  - ½ Tablespoon Coconut Oil
  - ¼ Cup Nutritional Yeast
  - Pink Himalayan Salt (to taste)
- ☐ **Tools**
  - Mixing Bowl
- ☐ **Method**

» Chop or tear kale to desired size.

» In mixing bowl, massage coconut oil thoroughly into kale.

» Add avocado. Mash with hands and mix thoroughly into kale.

» Add nutritional yeast. Mix well.

» Slice tomatoes in half.

» Add tomatoes and sliced onions to salad.

» Mix.

» Top with lemon juice and salt/pepper (to taste).

» Enjoy.

30. Southern Style Mango Cup

- ☐ **Ingredients**
  - 2 Mangos

- ½ Cup Apple Cider Vinegar
- Pink Himalayan Salt (to taste)
- ½ teaspoon Black Pepper
- ½ teaspoon Cayenne Pepper (optional)
- 2 tsp Chili lime Seasoning

☐ **Tools**

- Knife
- Cup or Container with a Lid

☐ **Method**

» Cut Mango into Spears or Chunks

» Place the mango spears into the cup

» Add Dry Ingredients

» Pour in Vinegar

» Shake up

» Enjoy!

Chapter 18

Bonus Recipes

<u>31. Nut Milk</u>

☐ **Ingredients**

- 1 Cup Cashews (or nut of choice)
- 2 Teaspoons Vanilla Extract
- 1 Teaspoon Cinnamon
- 1–2 Drops Stevia
- 2½ Cups Spring Water (use less water if you like your nut milk thick)

☐ **Tools**

- Nut Bag
- Blender
- Bowl
- Mason Jar with Cap

☐ **Method**

» Soak nut of choice for at least 1 hour in spring water. (If you can soak for longer, do so.)

» Combine drained nuts and all other ingredients in blender.

» Blend until smooth.

» Strain blend through nut bag into bowl.

» Be sure to squeeze all liquid into bowl.

» Pour nut milk out of bowl into mason jar with cap or another secure container.

» Enjoy!

32. Microwaveable Mug Bread (Low-Carb Friendly)

☐ **Ingredients**

- ¾ Cup Water
- ¼ Cup Ground Flaxseed
- 2 Dashes of Salt (to taste)
- 2 Tablespoons Psyllium Husk
- 1 Teaspoon Baking Flour
- 1 Cup Almond Flour
- 2 Teaspoons Cinnamon
- 1 Teaspoon Stevia
- ¼ Tablespoon Unsweetened Applesauce (optional)
- 1 Teaspoon Vegan Butter (per mug)

☐ **Tools**

- 2 Coffee Mugs
- Microwave
- Mixing Bowl
- Measuring Utensils

☐ **Method**

» Combine all dry ingredients.

» Mix thoroughly.

» Add water.

» Melt butter in mug; rub around mugs (prevents sticking).

» Split mix evenly into 2 coffee mugs.

» Microwave 80 seconds each (1000-watt microwave or higher).

» If you have lower powered microwave, adjust time.

» Slice evenly.

» Enjoy!